HOLISTIC HEALTH THROUGH CONSCIOUS THOUHGT

Overcoming Our Inner Self

Steven Hanner

ISBN: 979-8-89075-690-9

Contents

Introduction of the Author

Steven Hanner, nearing 60, has devoted much of his life to the repair industry, predominantly in troubleshooting. His extensive experience spans the Air Force, where he worked on aircraft electrical systems. After the military he repaired automotive vehicles for a few years, then spent the last three decades dedicated to office machine repairs such as printers, copiers, and scanners. A New Orleans native, Steven's only extended departure from the city was stationed in North Dakota during his time in the Air Force.

Steven's approach to health and fitness took an unforeseen turn approximately six and a half years ago. Initially, it wasn't a conscious decision; instead, he inadvertently stumbled upon a different path. As time passed, he realized his newfound techniques' simplicity and effectiveness, and pondered why more people were not embracing them. Intrigued, he delved into research, exploring the intricacies of exercise and the workings of the body, mind, and nervous system. Over years of piecing together information, he decided to share his insights by writing a book.

Before delving into health and fitness, Steven was unaware of the many remarkable benefits of exercise and how the whole thing works as an automated process to make our bodies stronger and more resilient. Damage is caused to the parts of our bodies used to make the physical exertions during exercise. This damage and subsequent repairs strengthen not only the individual parts of our body, but entire systems. In addition to all the muscles, bones, joints, ligaments, tendons, and more, our respiratory, and circulatory systems, among others, all benefit by this same process.

He also later determined that because of this strengthening, repetitious physical exertions will produce less damage each time, which diminishes this automatic process each time. This means our bodies can quickly adapt to repetitive exercises and the benefits that we initially get begin to diminish. Repetitive exercises limit and restrict our true capabilities of physical movement, so by engaging in the same exercise each day, we neglect many of the other parts of our body responsible for producing our physical movements. Suppose this automated process does not happen for long periods of time weather caused by inactivity or repetitive activity. In that case, all our body parts and systems work together to produce our physical movements and will decay from lack of use. These revelations surprised him and those he shared them with, as many people are oblivious to these aspects of exercise. Through his writings, he endeavors to demystify the effects of exercise on our bodies and minds, enabling readers to re-examine how they choose to live their lives.

Chapter 1: Balance

A natural balance between our bodies and minds was automatically obtained by thousands of generations of our ancestors living with nature, doing what they had to do to survive while eating only the natural foods available to them. Our bodies and minds were constructed by evolution to look and work the way they do, and they are still the same today. But everything else has changed in this artificial environment we've created. This has completely disrupted this balance. Our bodies and minds were designed to work together while interacting with the natural environment.

Thousands of years ago, our ancestors began to compete for food or shelter using mainly intelligence instead of physical attributes or instincts. We were the first and only species to harness fire, which allowed us to cook our food and gave us warmth and protection. Gathering around these fires probably greatly influenced the creation of our modern-day languages, which probably very quickly increased our intelligence because now we could share knowledge.

All recorded human history, which seems like a long time to us, is probably only about 10% of the human species' inhabitants. This meant that for most of their existence, our ancestors probably lived in small groups and hunted wild game or found other natural food sources. These mandatory activities in an ever-changing natural environment, such as droughts or floods, could affect these food sources. It often required them to relocate and adapt mentally and physically to new and different environments.

Many things quickly changed as we learned to domesticate animals and cultivate crops. This new abundance of food allowed people to live in larger groups in smaller areas, which led to the development of great cities and societies on an evolutionary scale in a very short time. This greatly began to influence many of our thoughts and behaviors. And the more intelligent we became, the faster this process continued. Rapid changes in our environments and thought processes began to have many adverse effects, causing great wars and the spread of major diseases.

We have made the most incredible technological advances in the last 50 to 100 years without realizing many of the negative impacts some of these advances, along with social pressures, have on us. It's almost impossible for any of us in our safe, comfortable artificial environments to imagine some of the challenges our hunter-gatherer ancestors had to endure daily.

Sometimes, we are told to walk more because our hunter-gatherer ancestors often walked. Yes, they did, but they didn't drive to a park and walk some lighted pathway wearing the same shoes every day at the same time. They were not just walking. They had to search for food and water or gather firewood. And when or if they found it, they had to figure out how to gather it up and carry it back. Over uneven terrain or up and down hills. In many different weather conditions while constantly being alert for threats or dangers in their environment. They had to learn their surroundings to remember how to return to where they came from. They had to figure out how to make their own tools, weapons, shelters, and anything else they needed. All these activities worked their minds and bodies together. There was also a strong sense of purpose and meaning to what they were doing. They had to do many of these things for their survival. Our ancestors probably used their brains much more than we do now because their lives depended on it.

The physical and mental challenges of someone running a marathon or on a treadmill is completely different from someone trying to chase down an animal to feed their family or running from a predator.

We use our intelligence and technology to make our lives easier and more comfortable, giving us much easier access to plenty of better-tasting foods. Not realizing that this could have negative effects, but it did. We began becoming unhealthy physically and mentally and still are. We were not designed to sit for hours in front of our TVs and computers or in our vehicles eating unnatural processed foods with little to no physical activity. So, to fix this problem, again, we used our intelligence and technology to come up with exercises.

What many of us do for exercise is completely unnatural. We were not designed to repeatedly lift the same heavyweights in the same direction with little to no purpose for doing it. This is because we have been conditioned to think that we must work on different parts of our bodies exclusively to achieve certain physical appearances or athletic performance goals. Then we have this idea that we need to do math problems and crossword puzzles to work our minds.

Our ancestors did not acquire intelligence from doing math problems and crossword puzzles, nor achieved their strength and speed from working out at a gym.

Our bodies and minds work optimally when used together as designed. This balance can never be completely restored, but engaging in more natural physical activities while eating natural healthy foods will bring us closer to fixing this balance instead of moving us further away.

Our minds still work the same as they did for most of our existence.

We don't seem to realize how far and fast our technological advances have removed us from the natural balance that has been occurring since the dawn of life on this planet.

This has had negative influences and consequences on our thoughts and behaviors as a society. This is a unique time in the history of our planet. For the first time, a species that not long ago harnessed fire now possesses the ability to extinguish all possible life.

Chapter 2: A Life of Quality

So many of us seem to care so much about how we look, what we own, or what other people are doing on social media. Little to no thought seems to go into our health and wellness or how this will affect our future.

Ensuring a high quality of life stands as an imperative pillar of our existence, for it serves as the bedrock upon which our long-term happiness is cultivated and nurtured. The pursuit of happiness, that elusive yet intrinsic human endeavor, finds its roots intertwined with the very fabric of our daily experiences and interactions. Each sunrise heralds the potential for new joys to be discovered, new passions to be kindled, and new paths to be explored in the grand tapestry of life.

Yet, what constitutes happiness is a deeply personal and subjective matter, varying from one individual to another and evolving with the shifting tides of time and circumstance. For some, it may be found in the warmth of cherished relationships, the embrace of loved ones who illuminate the darkest corners of our souls with their unwavering love and support. For others, it may manifest in the pursuit of knowledge and wisdom, the thrill of discovery and intellectual growth serving as guiding stars in the vast expanse of the unknown.

Indeed, the sources of our happiness are as diverse and multifaceted as the countless stars that adorn the night sky, each one shining with its own unique brilliance and allure. And just as the constellations shift and rearrange themselves over the course of the seasons, so too do our desires and aspirations ebb and flow with the passing of time.

In the pursuit of a fulfilling life, it is paramount that we remain attuned to the ever-changing landscape of our own desires and needs, adapting and evolving in accordance with the rhythm of our hearts and the cadence of our souls. For it is only by embracing the fluidity of our existence that we can hope to find true contentment and fulfillment, transcending the boundaries of expectation and convention to forge our own path towards happiness and self-actualization.

Thus, as we navigate the intricate tapestry of human experience, let us cherish the moments of joy and wonder that grace our lives, savoring each precious memory like a rare and precious jewel. And let us remember that true happiness lies not in the accumulation of material possessions or external accolades, but in the simple pleasures of everyday life—the laughter of loved ones, the beauty of nature, and the boundless potential that resides within each and every one of us.

With the advent of our modern technologies, we should be enjoying some of the finest quality of life in human history. We should be living longer, healthier happier lives, but something has gone wrong. The recent influence of TV shows and movies, along with the very recent ability to communicate instantly in multiple ways with massive numbers of people around the world has altered our very way of thinking in a very short period of time. All this has exponentially altered our perception, as a society, of what is generally accepted as morally right or wrong.

Just over 60 years ago even married couples could not be shown in the same bed on TV. The world and our societies were completely different. Due to the lack of 24/7 children's shows and video games, kids went outside and played real games, interacting with real people.

While walking, running, or bicycling, they explored and interacted with their environment. The reason kids were respectful to all adults is because of the consequences they knew they were going to receive. Where did we get this idea to quit spanking our children? This activity has been going on for a long time and has produced some of the finest generations of people in history.

In the fabric of our contemporary existence, a disconcerting pattern emerges: our once vibrant and promising youth seem to be losing their way amidst the ever-expanding realm of social media.

It's a troubling sight to behold as we witness a growing lack of respect and disregard for boundaries, coupled with concerning health issues like obesity. These young individuals, who have immersed themselves in the digital landscape for years, now appear to be shaping a narrative that raises profound questions about the caliber of future generations.

This troubling trajectory is poised to exacerbate further, driven by one of humanity's most influential and regrettably, perilous creations. The mega corporations orchestrating this phenomenon seem heedless to the repercussions their products inflict upon us and our children, prioritizing profit margins over the collective welfare of society. Their insatiable appetite for financial gain eclipses any semblance of moral responsibility, perpetuating a cycle of exploitation and disempowerment that threatens to undermine the very foundation of our social fabric.

All this has taken us so far off course that we may never be able to undo the damage that has been done. The only way we're going to begin to correct these problems is for each of us as individuals to consciously make the very important decisions that affect us and our children on a daily basis.

We have this perception that all our decisions are made consciously, but because of the way our minds really work, this is often not the case. We are all uniquely different based on our individual life experiences, but our minds all work the same way. We all have a subconscious and are unaware that this subconscious part of our mind makes most of our decisions automatically and immediately, with little to no conscious thought. Our subconscious is constructed by our life experiences, which are directly influenced by societal trends. This shapes our very way of thinking. We can overcome this naturally embedded programming and make conscious decisions, but first, we have to realize its existence and the power it can have over our daily decisions. In every situation, we can try to pause and think about what is actually happening, as opposed to what sometimes appears to be happening.

Each of our individual minds ultimately controls how we interpret everything in our lives, including our happiness.

Some of the activities we participate in are unknowingly based on the perception of the happiness we believe they will provide. This often unrealized pursuit of happiness can be heavily influenced by social pressures. We tend to follow the latest trends or acquire popular material things often just to win the approval of our peers.

Many of us go through our day-to-day lives seemingly unaware of how much many of our everyday choices can affect our quality of life, now and in the future. We usually tend to take the easier, more familiar paths as we go through our daily routines. The reason we find ourselves in the same coffee shop each morning or doing some other daily repetitive activity is due to this subconscious automatic process. Repetition leads to positive or negative habit formation.

Generations of social trends combined with individual life experiences and repetitive behaviors all influence the construction of our subconscious.

The decisions we make, whether consciously or subconsciously, wield a significant impact on our present and future well-being. It's crucial to acknowledge that these choices extend far beyond the realm of our immediate awareness, often influencing aspects of our lives that we may not fully grasp at the moment of decision-making. This is particularly evident in matters concerning our health and overall quality of life. Far too often, we find ourselves taking our health for granted, blissfully unaware of the potential consequences until it's too late. It's a common human tendency to prioritize short-term gratification over long-term sustainability, inadvertently neglecting the importance of preventative measures and holistic self-care practices. However, by cultivating a heightened sense of mindfulness and embracing proactive habits, we can mitigate the risks associated with such oversight, paving the way for a healthier and more fulfilling existence both now and in the days to come.

Why is it only after being diagnosed with some chronic disease or illness we choose to fight by changing our diets or lifestyles?

If these healthy choices had been made long ago, there's a good chance we wouldn't have gotten the disease, or it may not have affected us as severely. We all know we can much better fight off a disease if we're strong and healthy. And even if we get lucky and don't get any diseases, what do we want the final years of our lives to be like?

Do we want to be frail and weak, or suffer from mental decline, or have to spend the last years of our lives in a nursing home, or confined to a walker or wheelchair, often sick and in the hospital? If we sit around all day doing nothing but watching TV and eating unhealthy foods, some or all of these things will probably happen to us.

Wouldn't we rather be strong and confident and physically able to perform the task we enjoy? And mentally competent enough to do them. This would also allow us to maintain our independence.

Most of us want to live long, healthy, happy lives, physically and mentally, able to do the things we enjoy, often with friends or family, because these are the real things that can bring us the joy and happiness we all seek, along with the memories of these things to reflect on in our later years.

We go through our daily routines not realizing that putting a little more conscious thought into many of our daily choices can have a profound impact on our overall lifelong happiness.

The people who really love and care about us don't care how we look, what we own, or what we are posting on social media. What they really care about is that we're happy and healthy, and so should we.

Chapter 3: Health, Fitness and Everything in Between

Despite the availability of cutting-edge exercise equipment and a wealth of knowledge about human physiology, achieving and maintaining optimal health and fitness remains elusive for many individuals. This paradox is deeply rooted in our modern sedentary lifestyle, which has been exacerbated by the advent of technologies like television.

Approximately 50 years ago, as sedentary lifestyles became increasingly prevalent, the health and fitness industry emerged as a response to this growing concern. The rise of television, with its often-mind-numbing content, played a significant role in perpetuating sedentary habits. Coupled with the comfort of modern couches and recliners, television viewing has become a major contributor to a host of health issues, including pain, suffering, and premature death.

Today, the problem has only worsened with the proliferation of big-screen TVs and the phenomenon of binge-watching. Broadcasting companies capitalize on our sedentary habits by producing content that often highlights the darker aspects of human nature, thereby further entrenching negative behaviors. The alarming consequence is a population increasingly detached from physical activity, health-conscious behaviors, and, ultimately, optimal health and fitness.

In essence, despite the advancements in exercise science and equipment, our sedentary lifestyles, facilitated by technologies like television, have hindered our ability to achieve and sustain optimal health and fitness levels. Addressing this issue requires not only an individual commitment to physical activity but also societal changes that promote healthier lifestyles and discourage excessive sedentary behavior.

Health organizations are beginning to recognize the detrimental effects of inactivity on long-term physical and mental health. The sedentary lifestyle prevalent in modern society has prompted a reevaluation of the importance of physical activity in maintaining overall well-being.

It stands to reason that a moderate, consistent approach to physical activity is essential for promoting strength, mobility, and overall health throughout life. This approach emphasizes the importance of incorporating regular exercise into daily routines to enhance physical capabilities and support the performance of both mandatory and voluntary tasks.

However, the values of common sense and logic seem to be overshadowed by the profit-driven motives of the health and fitness industries. Rather than prioritizing genuine health and fitness goals, these industries often prioritize profit margins, leading to the proliferation of advertisements promoting unrealistic standards of physical fitness.

Many advertisements propagate the notion that achieving optimal fitness requires attaining the physique of a Greek god or gladiator, often through the use of technologically advanced exercise equipment. This artificial ideal creates unrealistic expectations and fosters a culture of quick-fix solutions and instant gratification.

It is concerning that some individuals are swayed by these misleading advertisements, purchasing machines and supplements in hopes of achieving overnight transformations. However, common sense dictates that such promises are likely scams, as the individuals featured in these advertisements likely did not attain their physique solely through the use of the advertised products.

In essence, while health organizations are beginning to recognize the importance of physical activity for long-term health, the health and fitness industries continue to prioritize profit over genuine well-being. Promoting a more balanced and realistic approach to fitness is essential to combatting the pervasive influence of unrealistic standards and promoting sustainable health practices.

The advertisements for exercise machines should not only focus on their fitness benefits but also acknowledge their potential alternative use as clothes hangers once their novelty wears off. This facetious remark highlights the disconnect between the lofty promises of these products and the reality of their usage.

Indeed, it begs the question: How did we stray so far from the true essence of health and fitness? Instead of emphasizing holistic well-being, the concept of fitness has been co-opted by social trends, which prioritize appearance over genuine health. This shift in perspective has created significant social pressures, leading individuals to pursue unrealistic standards of fitness at the expense of their well-being.

As a consequence, many individuals find themselves in a dangerous cycle, engaging in strenuous and often unnatural exercises on artificial equipment in pursuit of an idealized physique. This obsession with appearance-driven fitness not only increases the risk of injury but also undermines the foundational principles of health and well-being.

Moreover, there exists a misguided belief that health can be equated with the absence of illness and that any health issues can be remedied solely through medical intervention. This mindset is perpetuated by the pervasive influence of pharmaceutical advertisements, which promise quick fixes for a myriad of ailments, from physical appearance to mood enhancement and memory improvement.

The prevalence of such advertisements, often accompanied by offers of free samples, further perpetuates the illusion that these products hold the key to optimal health and well-being. However, the reality is far from the glossy promises of these advertisements, as evidenced by the excessive costs and dubious efficacy of many of these products.

In essence, the distortion of the concepts of health and fitness by social trends and commercial interests has led to a culture that prioritizes appearance over genuine well-being, perpetuating unrealistic standards and promoting harmful behaviors. Realigning our understanding of health and fitness to focus on holistic well-being is essential to counteracting these harmful influences and fostering a healthier society.

The notion that products are harmless because they are made with natural ingredients is often misguided, as evidenced by examples such as venomous snakes and poisonous mushrooms, which are entirely natural yet pose serious health risks. This highlights the fallacy of equating natural with safe, emphasizing the importance of critical thinking when evaluating health products and claims.

It is essential to recognize that years of physical inactivity and poor dietary habits cannot be remedied by pills or medications alone. Genuine improvement in fitness levels requires engaging in regular physical activity, which stimulates the body's natural repair processes and promotes overall well-being. This underscores the importance of adopting a holistic approach to health that prioritizes sustainable lifestyle changes over quick fixes or magic pills.

True health is not merely the absence of illness but encompasses physical capabilities and endurance. The ability to perform moderately difficult tasks, such as climbing a flight of stairs without becoming breathless, serves as a more accurate indicator of overall health and fitness.

Modern gadgets and expensive exercise equipment can create the illusion that achieving health and fitness goals requires external aids. However, it is essential to recognize that true health and fitness do not necessitate such tools. Instead, it requires understanding that the pursuit of fitness is deeply ingrained in societal perceptions, often influenced by media portrayals of muscular individuals. These repetitive images, reinforced over the years, shape our subconscious associations with health and fitness, leading to the misconception that achieving a specific physique is necessary for optimal health.

In reality, individuals come in diverse shapes and sizes, each with unique motivations and goals. Embracing this diversity and understanding that health and fitness are multifaceted concepts can help dispel the illusion of a one-size-fits-all approach to physical well-being. By redefining our understanding of health and fitness and embracing sustainable lifestyle habits, we can cultivate a more inclusive and realistic approach to promoting overall well-being for all individuals.

The prevalence of modern-day charlatans and snake oil salesmen underscores the need for a deeper understanding of how our minds function. These individuals, who have existed for centuries, now wield almost unlimited influence in a globalized society. Their manipulation tactics prey on our vulnerabilities, distorting our perceptions of health and fitness and steering us towards unsustainable and often harmful methods of achieving our goals.

The negative impact of this manipulation is evident in the choices we make regarding our health and fitness. In our increasingly sedentary and artificial environment, we are bombarded with messages that prioritize superficial physical appearances over holistic well-being. This narrow focus on aesthetics leads us astray from common sense principles, such as skepticism towards offers that seem too good to be true.

To truly reap the benefits of health and fitness, we must shift away from this superficial narrative and return to fundamental principles grounded in common sense. A moderate, long-term, and consistent approach is essential for nurturing both our physical bodies and our mental well-being throughout our lifetimes. This entails recognizing that health encompasses more than just outward appearances and requires a holistic understanding of our bodies and minds.

By embracing these common-sense principles and rejecting the allure of quick fixes and unrealistic promises, we can reclaim control over our health and fitness goals. Only then can we cultivate a lifestyle that fosters genuine strength, resilience, and longevity, both physically and mentally.

Chapter 4: The Problem with Exercise

The realm of exercise science has long been dominated by studies that focus on controlled, artificial activities like aerobic or strength training routines. While these studies have undoubtedly contributed valuable insights into the physiological effects of exercise, they may inadvertently overlook the profound benefits of natural physical activities in promoting holistic health and well-being.

Natural physical activities encompass a wide range of movements that are deeply ingrained in human culture and history. From playing physically demanding sports to participating in extreme dance contests, these activities offer unique advantages that extend beyond the scope of traditional exercise routines. Unlike the repetitive motions often associated with structured workouts, natural physical activities involve dynamic movements that engage multiple muscle groups, challenge coordination and balance, and stimulate cognitive functions such as decision-making and spatial awareness.

One of the distinguishing features of natural physical activities is their ability to mimic real-life movements and scenarios. For example, playing a game of soccer requires participants to sprint, jump, kick, and pivot, all while making split-second decisions in response to changing circumstances on the field. Similarly, engaging in a dance competition involves fluid movements, intricate footwork, and precise timing, demanding both physical agility and mental acuity.

Moreover, natural physical activities foster a sense of camaraderie and social connection that is often lacking in solitary exercise routines. Whether it's playing on a team, dancing in a group, or engaging in outdoor recreational activities with friends and family, these experiences promote social bonding, cooperation, and mutual support. The social aspect of natural physical activities not only enhances motivation and enjoyment but also contributes to overall well-being by reducing feelings of loneliness and isolation.

In addition to their physical and social benefits, natural physical activities have been shown to have a positive impact on mental health and emotional well-being. The immersive nature of activities like sports and dance allows individuals to experience a state of flow characterized by deep concentration, heightened focus, and a sense of timelessness. This state of flow has been associated with increased feelings of happiness, fulfillment, and overall life satisfaction.

Furthermore, natural physical activities provide a welcome respite from the stresses and pressures of everyday life. Engaging in a challenging game or exhilarating dance performance offers a temporary escape from worries and anxieties, allowing individuals to recharge and rejuvenate both mentally and physically. The sense of accomplishment and satisfaction that comes from mastering a new skill or achieving a personal best can boost self-esteem and confidence, fostering a positive mindset and outlook on life.

Despite the myriad benefits of natural physical activities, they are often overlooked or undervalued in the realm of exercise science. The focus on controlled, artificial activities in research and public health initiatives may perpetuate the misconception that exercise is synonymous with structured workouts in a gym setting. However, by recognizing the unique advantages of natural physical activities and incorporating them into exercise recommendations and interventions, we can promote a more diverse and inclusive approach to fitness that prioritizes enjoyment, social connection, and overall well-being.

Furthermore, the motivations driving individuals to engage in natural physical activities can vary widely and may have different impacts on their overall well-being. For example, someone participating in a team sport may derive motivation from camaraderie, competition, and the pursuit of shared goals, whereas an individual engaging in an extreme dance contest may be driven by personal expression, creativity, and the thrill of performance.

Comparing the effects of natural physical activities to structured exercise routines could provide valuable insights into the holistic benefits of movement. It may reveal how factors such as social interaction, enjoyment, and varied movement patterns influence physical and mental health outcomes.

Additionally, recognizing the diverse motivations behind physical activity participation can inform the development of more tailored and engaging exercise programs that cater to individual preferences and goals. By embracing a broader perspective on movement and exercise, researchers and practitioners can better support individuals in achieving optimal health and well-being across the lifespan.

Our understanding of the profound benefits of exercise is evolving alongside our comprehension of the intricate workings of the human body and mind. Overlooked for years, the fascia system, a network of connective tissue enveloping our organs, muscles, and cells, is emerging as a pivotal player in physical movement. Collaborating with muscles, it facilitates fluid motion and, when healthy, enables freedom of movement while safeguarding against pain and restriction.

Similarly, the enigmatic nature of our brains continues to intrigue professionals. While we possess both conscious and subconscious realms, it's the latter that orchestrates the majority of our actions, often beyond our conscious awareness. This subconscious control influences the activities we engage in daily, including exercise.

Contrary to common understanding, exercise operates through a series of natural, automated processes that enhance our physical resilience. When we engage in physical exertion, muscle contractions initiate micro-damage across various bodily structures. However, this damage serves as a catalyst for repair and growth. Not only do muscles strengthen, but bones also fortify, becoming more resistant to fractures. Additionally, joints, ligaments, and tendons benefit, supported by improvements in circulatory, respiratory, immune, and endocrine systems.

This repair process is driven by the release of chemicals and hormones like Irisin, which trigger cascades of physiological responses. Enhanced heart rate and breathing increase oxygen delivery to cells, expediting waste removal. Consequently, the lungs and heart become stronger and more efficient while blood vessels maintain elasticity. These adaptations fuel the proliferation and efficiency of mitochondria within cells, optimizing energy production and raising VO2 max, all while generating internal warmth. Thus, exercise, once seen as merely physical exertion, emerges as a sophisticated interplay of bodily systems, fostering strength, resilience, and vitality from within.

The paradox of exercise lies in its undeniable benefits contrasted with the struggle many face in incorporating it into their lives consistently. Despite the well-documented advantages of exercise, such as improved physical health, mental well-being, and resilience, a significant portion of the population fails to engage in regular physical activity.

The cyclical pattern observed in gyms, with a surge of new members at the start of the year followed by a return to familiar faces after a few weeks or months, highlights the challenge of maintaining exercise habits. The phenomenon of New Year's resolutions reflects a desire for change, yet the transient nature of motivation often leads to abandoned goals.

Part of the issue lies in the artificial nature of exercise itself. Invented to counteract the sedentary lifestyles characteristic of modern society, exercise can feel disconnected from our natural inclinations. Unlike other species, we engage in physical activities devoid of inherent meaning or purpose, which may deter long-term adherence.

Moreover, individual preferences and past experiences influence exercise choices. Runners run, weightlifters lift weights, and cyclists cycle, reflecting a tendency to gravitate towards familiar activities. While initially, the novelty of starting a new exercise regimen or revisiting past routines may evoke feelings of excitement and optimism, these sentiments often wane over time.

The decline in motivation and subsequent cessation of exercise can trigger feelings of disappointment and self-doubt. Individuals may interpret their inability to maintain consistency as a lack of discipline or willpower, exacerbating negative emotions and perpetuating the cycle of inactivity.

Addressing the challenge of exercise adherence requires a multifaceted approach. Recognizing the artificial nature of exercise and aligning activities with personal interests and values can enhance motivation and long-term engagement. Additionally, fostering a supportive environment and reframing setbacks as opportunities for growth can mitigate feelings of failure and promote resilience in pursuit of fitness goals. Ultimately, cultivating a positive mindset and adopting sustainable habits are key to overcoming the barriers to regular physical activity and unlocking the transformative potential of exercise.

The concept of exercise, while intended to promote health and well-being, paradoxically presents challenges that stem from its artificial nature and repetitive characteristics.

Our subconscious mind not only influences the choice of exercises but also dictates the execution of repetitive movements inherent in many exercise routines. Despite the variety of exercises available, individuals often find themselves defaulting to the same repetitive actions, such as lifting weights in a specific direction for a set duration. These movements, though seemingly beneficial, are unnatural and fail to mimic the diverse range of movements our bodies are designed for.

Moreover, the tendency to engage in repetitive exercises limits the full potential of physical movement and neglects the holistic needs of the body. While certain muscle groups may strengthen from repetitive exercises, other parts of the body responsible for producing movement may become neglected and atrophy due to lack of use. This contradicts the perceived intention of exercise, which is often undertaken to prevent physical deterioration.

Furthermore, the repetitive nature of exercise can lead to disengagement of the conscious mind, resulting in boredom and decreased motivation. Similar to how individuals tire of hearing the same songs or watching the same movies repeatedly, engaging in repetitive exercises may trigger a similar response. As a result, individuals may abandon these exercises for extended periods, further hindering their overall physical activity levels.

Ultimately, the very tool intended to encourage movement and improve health may inadvertently contribute to stagnation and decreased physical activity. Recognizing the limitations of repetitive exercises and exploring alternative forms of movement that embrace diversity and engagement may offer a more sustainable approach to promoting overall well-being.

The spectrum of physical activities available to maintain fitness extends far beyond traditional repetitive exercises, encompassing natural and engaging pursuits that benefit both body and mind.

Yoga and Pilates stand out as alternatives to repetitive exercises, offering holistic approaches to fitness that prioritize flexibility, strength, and mindfulness. While these practices can become routine, their emphasis on breath control, body awareness, and fluid movements sets them apart from traditional gym routines. Furthermore, engaging in physical games with children or peers injects an element of playfulness and social interaction into fitness activities, enhancing enjoyment and motivation.

Looking beyond structured exercises, natural physical activities such as playing games and dancing emerge as timeless practices rooted in human history. These activities engage the body and mind holistically, requiring skills, strategies, and teamwork while providing enjoyment and fulfillment. Unlike the monotony of traditional exercise routines, playing and dancing tap into our innate instincts for movement and social interaction, promoting overall well-being in a natural and meaningful way.

Despite the wealth of evidence supporting the benefits of natural physical activities, many studies on exercise fail to consider these factors comprehensively. The largest study ever conducted, spanning hundreds of millions of people over thousands of years, underscores the profound impact of purposeful and meaningful physical activities on our bodies and minds. By embracing the diversity of natural physical activities, individuals can cultivate a more balanced and fulfilling approach to fitness that aligns with our evolutionary heritage and enhances overall health and well-being.

Chapter 5: Eating Healthy

For eons, the quest for sustenance has been the primary driving force behind the evolution of life on Earth. Within this intricate dance of survival, those organisms capable of securing food thrived, passing on their advantageous traits to subsequent generations. From the smallest microbe to the mightiest predator, the ability to procure nourishment dictated an organism's fate.

Plants, harnessing the sun's energy through photosynthesis, provided the foundation of this intricate web of life. Their green leaves, bathed in sunlight, synthesized sugars and other vital nutrients, initiating a chain reaction that sustained entire ecosystems. Animals, in turn, feasted upon these plant-based energies, while others pursued fellow creatures for sustenance. Each species, sculpted by millennia of natural selection, possessed a unique set of attributes finely tuned for survival in their respective niches.

This symbiotic relationship between predator and prey, herbivores and plants, fostered a delicate equilibrium in nature. The relentless pressure of natural selection ensured that only the fittest survived, maintaining the vigor and resilience of populations over time. The interplay of physical prowess and cognitive acumen is honed through generations of evolutionary trial and error.

However, this harmonious rhythm was disrupted with the advent of a relatively new player on the evolutionary stage: Homo sapiens. Approximately 12,000 years ago, these early humans embarked on a transformative journey, one that would forever alter the course of history. Armed with intellect and innovation, they began to manipulate their environment in unprecedented ways.

The transition from hunter-gatherer societies to settled agricultural communities marked a pivotal turning point in human history. Through cultivation and domestication, humans gained unprecedented control over their food sources, reshaping landscapes and ecosystems in the process. No longer bound by the constraints of foraging, they could now cultivate crops and raise livestock, fundamentally altering the dynamics of food acquisition.

This agricultural revolution, while heralding newfound stability and abundance for human populations, also brought about profound consequences. The once-natural balance of ecosystems was disrupted as humans exerted their influence on a global scale. Species were domesticated, landscapes transformed, and biodiversity diminished as agriculture became increasingly intensive.

Yet, even as the modern world grapples with the ramifications of this paradigm shift, the fundamental truth remains unchanged: food and the pursuit thereof, continue to shape the trajectory of life on Earth. From the microscopic to the monumental, the quest for sustenance remains the driving force of evolution, an eternal testament to the enduring power of nature's design.

The natural world operates on a delicate balance, sculpted by the relentless forces of natural selection. Each organism plays a vital role, finely tuned to its environment through generations of evolutionary refinement. Plants and animals, in their natural habitats, are subject to the unyielding pressures of survival, resulting in ecosystems that are finely tuned to maintain health and vigor.

Through the domestication of animals and the cultivation of crops, humans exerted their influence on the very fabric of life itself. By selectively breeding plants and animals for desired traits, humans inadvertently skewed the natural evolutionary processes, leading to unforeseen consequences for both our food sources and the ecosystems that support them.

This manipulation of nature gave rise to a reliance on artificial means of food production. As the demand for sustenance grew alongside human populations, the quest for efficiency led to the emergence of processed food. By distilling nutrients into easily accessible forms, humans sought to meet the ever-increasing demand for food with minimal effort.

However, this quest for convenience came at a steep cost. The proliferation of processed foods brought with it a myriad of unforeseen health consequences, as diets rich in artificial additives and preservatives began to take their toll on human health. Moreover, the industrialization of agriculture led to the degradation of ecosystems, as monoculture farming and intensive livestock production wreaked havoc on the environment.

As human societies transitioned from small hunter-gatherer groups to larger settlements and civilizations, the demand for food skyrocketed. Animals were confined to pens and cages, while vast expanses of land were cleared for agriculture, further exacerbating the strain on natural resources.

In this relentless pursuit of abundance, humanity found itself locked in a vicious cycle of overconsumption and environmental degradation. The once-balanced ecosystems of old gave way to a landscape dominated by human activity, where the very foundations of life were reshaped to suit our needs.

Yet, even as the consequences of our actions reverberate throughout the natural world, the inherent resilience of life endures. In the face of adversity, nature has a remarkable ability to adapt and evolve, offering hope for a future where harmony between humankind and the environment can once again be restored.

The shift towards reliance on unnatural food sources marked a pivotal moment in human history, not only in terms of sustenance but also in the socio-economic dynamics of societies. With the emergence of processed foods and industrialized agriculture, food ceased to be solely a means of survival; it transformed into a symbol of wealth and status, conferring upon individuals the power to influence and control.

In this new paradigm, those who possessed abundant food resources wielded considerable influence within their communities. The accumulation of food became a measure of prosperity, affording individuals the means to assert dominance and ascend to positions of power. Thus, the stage was set for the birth of the politician, a figure tasked with managing the distribution of resources and navigating the complexities of societal hierarchy.

However, with the consolidation of power came the inevitable specter of corruption. As individuals vied for control over increasingly valuable food resources, the temptation to exploit their positions for personal gain became all too prevalent. Nepotism, bribery, and deceit became endemic as those in positions of authority sought to consolidate their power and influence at the expense of the common good.

Moreover, the introduction of marketplaces and the practice of bartering further fueled the fires of greed and avarice. No longer bound by the constraints of traditional subsistence farming, individuals now had the opportunity to amass wealth through trade and commerce. Yet, with this newfound prosperity came the insidious influence of money, a force that would irrevocably alter the fabric of society.

As the pursuit of wealth became increasingly paramount, the values of community and cooperation began to erode. Money, with its promise of power and prestige, emerged as the new driving force behind human interactions, eclipsing the once-central role of food in sustaining social cohesion. The insatiable desire for wealth gave rise to a culture of exploitation and inequality, where the few wielded disproportionate influence over the lives of the many.

In this brave new world, the pursuit of profit supplanted the pursuit of sustenance as the primary motivator of human behavior. Communities and civilizations were reshaped by this relentless pursuit of wealth, as individuals clamored to secure their place within the hierarchy of power. Humanity lost sight of the fundamental values that once bound us together, leaving in its wake a legacy of greed, inequality, and moral decay.

The advancements in food production ushered in by industrialization and agricultural innovation revolutionized human society, granting us the unprecedented ability to sustain large populations and even armies. With these newfound capabilities, nations began to amass vast reserves of food, transforming it into a potent weapon of war and a tool of geopolitical dominance.

However, the very products of our unnatural societies—processed foods laden with artificial additives and preservatives—bore unforeseen consequences. As nations engaged in conflicts over resources and territory, food became a strategic asset, wielded to devastating effects on the battlefield. Wars fought over control of food-producing regions or access to vital agricultural resources ravaged entire populations, leaving devastation in their wake.

Furthermore, the rapid globalization facilitated by modern trade networks inadvertently facilitated the spread of infectious diseases. Unnatural food products, often produced in unsanitary conditions or contaminated with harmful pathogens, became vectors for the transmission of illness on a global scale. The convergence of densely populated urban centers and widespread food distribution networks created fertile ground for the proliferation of epidemics, wreaking havoc on human populations worldwide.

Ironically, the very efforts aimed at increasing food availability often yielded unintended consequences. While industrialized agriculture succeeded in producing vast quantities of food, its reliance on monoculture farming and chemical inputs led to environmental degradation and loss of biodiversity. Moreover, the abundance of processed foods, high in calories but low in nutritional value, contributed to a global epidemic of obesity and related health problems.

Yet, amidst this paradox of plenty, millions around the world still grapple with hunger and malnutrition. The unequal distribution of resources and the inefficiencies of food production and distribution systems mean that while some regions enjoy abundance, others languish in deprivation. Starvation, a silent scourge often overshadowed by the specter of armed conflict, remains a potent weapon used by governments and insurgent groups alike to control populations and exert influence over rival factions.

In this complex web of human existence, food serves as both a source of sustenance and a catalyst for conflict. The unintended consequences of our relentless pursuit of progress have reshaped the very fabric of society, leaving a trail of devastation in their wake. Yet, amidst the chaos and uncertainty, there remains hope for a more equitable and sustainable future—one where food is no longer a weapon of war but a shared resource that nourishes and sustains all of humanity.

The march of commercial industries, driven by profit and efficiency, has brought our natural environment to the brink of collapse. Nowhere is this more evident than in the oceans, where overfishing and environmental degradation threaten the very foundations of marine ecosystems. Once-abundant natural food sources are rapidly dwindling, pushed to the brink of extinction by industrial-scale exploitation. If this trend continues unchecked, the consequences could be catastrophic, with the potential for widespread starvation and ecosystem collapse looming large on the horizon.

Yet, even as we stand on the precipice of this environmental crisis, our attempts to rectify the situation often seem to exacerbate the problem. Time and again, our reliance on intelligence and technology to solve complex problems has backfired, leading to unintended consequences and unforeseen challenges. The pursuit of convenience and efficiency has led us down a perilous path, where the solutions we devise only serve to deepen the underlying issues.

Nowhere is this more evident than in the realm of processed foods. These modern marvels of food engineering, with their enticing flavors and addictive qualities, have inundated our diets with unhealthy, high-calorie fare. Marketed relentlessly to consumers, especially children, these foods represent a stark departure from the natural, nutrient-dense diets our bodies evolved to consume.

In a desperate attempt to mitigate the health consequences of our dietary choices, we have resorted to extreme measures. Fad diets, artificial sweeteners, and medications offer temporary reprieves from the consequences of our indulgence, but they fail to address the root cause of the problem: our dysfunctional relationship with food.

From sugary donuts in the workplace to late-night drive-thru cravings, the temptation to indulge in unhealthy foods is ever-present. Yet, the consequences of these choices extend far beyond our waistlines. Our health, our well-being, and the health of the planet are all intrinsically linked to the foods we consume.

In a world inundated with choice, the decision of what to eat has never been more important. Yet, for many, the allure of convenience and instant gratification often outweighs the consideration of long-term health consequences. Breaking free from this cycle of unhealthy eating requires a fundamental shift in mindset, one that prioritizes nourishment and sustainability over convenience and indulgence.

Ultimately, the choices we make about food are a reflection of our values and priorities as a society. If we are to address the myriad challenges facing our food system, we must first recognize the interconnectedness of our choices and their consequences. Only then can we begin to forge a path towards a healthier, more sustainable future for ourselves and the planet.

In our modern world, eating healthy is often portrayed as a daunting task, but the real challenge lies in overcoming the deeply ingrained subconscious patterns that dictate our food choices. Generations of exposure to marketing tactics, coupled with the omnipresence and convenience of processed foods, have led us to believe that these foods are not only acceptable but preferable.

To reclaim our health and well-being, we must endeavor to return to a diet comprised of the natural foods that sustained our ancestors. Fresh meats, fruits, vegetables, nuts, and seeds, prepared simply through baking or grilling, offer a return to the basics of nourishment. By eschewing the myriad seasonings, sauces, and dressings that inundate modern diets, we can reconnect with the inherent flavors and nutritional benefits of whole foods.

A crucial aspect of eating healthily is understanding what we're putting into our bodies. Each food item should contain only one ingredient, devoid of the lengthy lists of unpronounceable additives and preservatives that characterize processed foods. By opting for foods with simple, recognizable ingredients, we can regain control over our diets and prioritize our health and well-being.

Variety is key when it comes to eating healthily. By incorporating a diverse array of natural foods into our diets, we can ensure that our bodies receive the full spectrum of nutrients they need to thrive. Our bodies were designed to digest and metabolize these foods, as they have been a staple of the human diet throughout our evolutionary history.

In essence, eating healthily is not about adhering to strict diets or depriving ourselves of the foods we enjoy. Rather, it is about returning to a more natural way of eating, one that honors the inherent wisdom of our bodies and the bounty of the earth. By embracing whole, unprocessed foods and listening to our bodies' signals of hunger and satiety, we can forge a path toward optimal health and vitality.

Our gut microbiome, a complex ecosystem of bacteria residing in our digestive tract, plays a fundamental role in our overall health and well-being. These microorganisms automatically adapt to the foods we consume, with different types of bacteria specializing in the digestion of specific nutrients. By nourishing our bodies with natural, healthy foods, we not only encourage the growth of beneficial bacteria but also tap into an ancient symbiotic relationship that has supported human digestion for centuries.

Indeed, the foods we eat have a profound impact on our gut microbiome, shaping its composition and function. Natural, nutrient-dense foods provide the necessary fuel for the growth and proliferation of beneficial bacteria, which in turn aid in the digestion and absorption of essential nutrients. Over time, as we consistently consume healthy foods, our gut microbiome becomes attuned to processing these foods efficiently, creating cravings for wholesome, natural flavors while diminishing the allure of processed, unhealthy options.

However, eating healthy is just one piece of the puzzle when it comes to maintaining optimal digestive health. Our digestive system operates in concert with numerous other bodily systems, each relying on the health and functionality of the others to operate optimally. Physical activity, for example, not only improves the efficiency of our digestive system but also increases the demand for energy, prompting the body to burn calories and regulate glucose levels more effectively.

Furthermore, the natural vitamins and minerals found in healthy foods are absorbed more efficiently when the body is engaged in physical activity, aiding in the repair and maintenance of all bodily systems. This holistic approach to health recognizes the interconnectedness of our bodily systems and emphasizes the importance of nurturing each component to achieve overall well-being.

In considering our approach to nutrition and health, it's important to look to our ancestors for guidance. For thousands of years, our predecessors relied on instinct and physical activity to maintain their health and vitality. They did not adhere to rigid dietary guidelines or schedules but instead ate according to the rhythms of nature, fueling their bodies with the foods they could find or procure through physical exertion.

Intermediate fasting, a practice that mimics the natural patterns of food availability experienced by our ancestors, may indeed hold benefits for modern health. By embracing this ancient practice, we can tap into our body's innate ability to regulate hunger and metabolism, promoting greater overall health and well-being.

Thus, achieving optimal health requires a holistic approach that considers the interconnectedness of our bodily systems and embraces the natural rhythms of nutrition and physical activity. By nourishing our bodies with wholesome, natural foods and engaging in regular exercise, we can support the health and functionality of our digestive system and promote overall vitality and longevity.

Chapter 6: Learning and Unlearning

Learning is an essential aspect of human existence, allowing us to expand our horizons, develop new skills, and evolve as individuals. It's the process through which we acquire knowledge, skills, behaviors, and attitudes, ultimately shaping our understanding of the world and our place within it.

One fundamental truth about learning is its boundless nature. There's no limit to the amount of knowledge or skills we can accumulate over a lifetime. From mastering new languages to acquiring expertise in various fields, the potential for learning seems limitless. This capacity to learn is a remarkable aspect of human cognition, enabling us to adapt, innovate, and thrive in diverse environments.

However, despite our remarkable ability to absorb information and acquire new skills, there's a curious paradox: we often struggle to learn from our past mistakes. While we have the capability to gather vast amounts of knowledge and experience, applying these lessons to avoid repeating errors can be challenging. This cognitive bias highlights the complexity of human behavior and decision-making processes as we struggle with factors like ego, emotions, and entrenched habits.

In today's digital age, access to information has reached unprecedented levels. With the internet and smartphones, we carry the sum of human knowledge in our pockets, akin to having a vast library at our fingertips. Yet, despite this wealth of resources, many people squander their time on trivial pursuits like celebrity gossip or sports updates, neglecting the transformative potential of education and self-improvement.

When we think of learning, we often associate it with formal education, such as attending schools or classrooms. While structured learning environments play a crucial role in imparting knowledge and skills, true learning extends far beyond these boundaries. Life itself is a classroom, offering lessons through experiences, challenges, and interactions with others. This experiential learning is particularly impactful, as it provides insights that textbooks and lectures cannot fully convey.

Younger individuals, though often encouraged to prioritize education, may not fully grasp its significance until they accumulate life experiences. The wisdom gained from various situations, overcoming obstacles, and interacting with diverse perspectives enriches our understanding of the world and fosters personal growth.

Moreover, learning isn't solely about intellectual pursuits; it also has practical implications for our livelihoods and well-being. Acquiring specialized skills and knowledge can enhance our employability, opening doors to diverse career opportunities. Additionally, the demands of our daily work, along with financial achievements and interpersonal relationships, shape our identities and lifestyles over time.

Learning is a multifaceted process that permeates every aspect of human existence. It's not just about acquiring facts and figures but also about cultivating curiosity, critical thinking, and adaptability. By embracing a lifelong commitment to learning, we empower ourselves to deal with life's complexities, fulfill our potential, and contribute meaningfully to the world around us.

Learning is not confined to the walls of classrooms or the structured curriculum of formal education; it can emerge from a myriad of sources, each offering unique opportunities for growth and enrichment. One of the most accessible and expansive reservoirs of knowledge lies within the boundless expanse of the internet. Here, a wealth of resources awaits, from digital libraries brimming with books and articles to an array of educational videos spanning every conceivable topic.

Among these resources, reading occupies a special place, distinguished by its ability to stimulate the imagination and engage the mind in the process of active interpretation. Unlike passive forms of media like television or videos, reading requires the reader to mentally construct images, scenarios, and characters, fostering deeper comprehension and retention of information. Through reading, we embark on journeys of discovery, traversing the landscapes of history, science, literature, and beyond, all while exercising our cognitive faculties and expanding our horizons.

Moreover, learning extends beyond the acquisition of knowledge; it encompasses the development of physical skills that engage both the body and mind in tandem. Whether mastering a musical instrument, honing athletic abilities, or cultivating artisanal craftsmanship, learning new physical skills offers a holistic form of education that integrates cognitive, motor, and sensory functions. This fusion of mental and physical engagement not only enhances our dexterity and coordination but also promotes mental agility and creative problem-solving.

In the pursuit of learning, the emphasis should always be on the quality of knowledge and skills acquired rather than the sheer quantity of information amassed. A discerning approach to learning ensures that we prioritize depth over breadth, delving into subjects with curiosity, critical inquiry, and a commitment to mastery. By focusing on the quality of learning experiences, we cultivate a nuanced understanding of complex concepts, develop expertise in areas of interest, and foster a lifelong passion for intellectual growth.

Promoting the endeavor of learning as a vital lifelong pursuit is essential for fostering personal development, intellectual curiosity, and societal progress. Encouraging individuals to embrace learning as an ongoing journey instills a sense of agency, self-improvement, and adaptability in the face of change. Whether through formal education, self-directed study, hands-on experiences, or interactions with diverse communities, the pursuit of knowledge and skill acquisition enriches our lives, broadens our perspectives, and empowers us to face the world with confidence and competence.

Before we ever step into a classroom or crack open a book, our minds are already hard at work, laying the groundwork for learning through a process that begins long before conscious awareness takes hold. From the moment of birth, our subconscious begins its meticulous compilation of a vast repository of knowledge and skills, shaping the very essence of who we are and how we interact with the world.

At the dawn of our existence, we embark on a journey of discovery, mastering the intricate art of movement through the acquisition of motor skills. This foundational learning process unfolds instinctively as we learn how to roll over, crawl, balance, and eventually walk and run. These initial forays into physicality lay the groundwork for all subsequent movements, setting the stage for a lifetime of physical mastery.

The beauty of this process lies in its integration into our being. The subconscious mind orchestrates these movements effortlessly, allowing our conscious faculties to remain attuned to the myriad stimuli of our surroundings. This innate ability to perform complex actions without conscious awareness, known as procedural memory, is a testament to the remarkable efficiency of the human brain.

Behind the scenes, a symphony of neural activity unfolds as over 600 muscles engage in a delicate dance of contraction and release, guided by the unseen hand of our subconscious. The complexity of these interactions, choreographed with precision against the backdrop of gravity, far exceeds the capacity of our conscious minds to comprehend or control.

This process of learning and memory formation is driven by the principles of neuroplasticity, wherein the brain undergoes structural and functional changes in response to repeated stimuli. Through the repetition of tasks and activities, new neural connections are forged and reinforced, giving rise to distinct clusters of neurons dedicated to specific skills and memories.

Indeed, it's not just physical skills that are etched into our neural architecture through this process; every memory, whether consciously acquired or subconsciously absorbed, is stored in our brain's neural networks. These collections of neurons serve as the custodians of our abilities and experiences, faithfully preserving our very existence.

In essence, the journey of learning begins long before we are even aware of it, as our subconscious mind lays the foundation for a lifetime of growth and discovery. From the primal rhythms of movement to the depths of our most cherished memories, the workings of the brain shape the very essence of our being, guiding us on a journey of self-discovery and transformation.

Throughout our lives, we are engaged in a constant process of subconscious learning that far surpasses our conscious comprehension. Much of this learning occurs beneath the surface of awareness as our brains effortlessly absorb and assimilate a wealth of information from our everyday experiences.

Communication, for instance, is a multifaceted endeavor that involves far more than the mere exchange of words. In addition to verbal language, we convey meaning through mannerisms, body language, facial expressions, and vocal inflections. Each of these elements is orchestrated by our neural networks, which coordinate the precise contractions of muscles to produce gestures, expressions, and tones that convey our thoughts and emotions.

Consider the complexity involved in the production and comprehension of speech. Every word we utter, along with its accompanying nuances of regional accents and intonations, is effortlessly executed by our brains, which activate the appropriate groups of neurons to instigate movements of our vocal apparatus. Simultaneously, other neural circuits decode the sounds we hear, allowing us to comprehend and interpret spoken language with remarkable speed and accuracy.

This integration of motor and sensory processes enables us to engage in conversations while simultaneously performing other tasks, a testament to the efficiency of our subconscious learning mechanisms. Even seemingly mundane activities, such as learning the steps of a new dance or memorizing the lyrics of a song, are facilitated by this automatic encoding of muscle contractions into procedural memory.

Underlying this process is the phenomenon of neuroplasticity, the brain's remarkable ability to reorganize and adapt in response to experience. Neuroplasticity ensures that the connections between neurons are continuously refined and strengthened, enabling the acquisition and retention of new skills and knowledge. Just as our bodies automatically regulate essential functions like breathing and heartbeat, neuroplasticity operates as an automatic system, engaging only when necessary to facilitate learning and adaptation.

The vast majority of our learning occurs beneath the surface of conscious awareness, driven by the automatic processes of our brain. From the subtle nuances of nonverbal communication to the intricate mechanics of language production, our subconscious mind serves as a silent but powerful engine of learning, constantly shaping our understanding of the world and our interactions within it.

Learning is a dynamic process that shapes our brains and behaviors, yet it's often easier to engage in familiar activities than to embark on new learning endeavors. Just as physical exercise is essential for maintaining optimal bodily function, engaging in novel experiences and learning new skills is crucial for the health and vitality of our brains.

The process of constructing and strengthening neural connections, known as neuroplasticity, is akin to a workout for our brains. Just as physical activity benefits all cells in the body, stimulating neuroplasticity through learning not only reinforces new connections but also enhances the overall function of the brain. However, like muscles that atrophy from lack of use, the brain's capacity for neuroplasticity can decline if not regularly exercised through learning and novel experiences.

Consider the seemingly mundane task of walking to the refrigerator. What may appear as a simple action actually involves a complex series of coordinated muscle contractions orchestrated by the brain to propel us forward while simultaneously stabilizing our body. This routine, ingrained through repetition, becomes second nature, requiring minimal conscious effort to execute.

Indeed, our daily lives are filled with routines and patterns that our subconscious mind readily assumes control of, freeing our conscious mind for other tasks. However, the downside of this automation is that it can lead to a lack of stimulation for the brain, potentially resulting in feelings of boredom or even depression. Without the challenge of learning and adaptation, our brains may stagnate, deprived of the variety and novelty that foster growth and resilience.

In contrast to the structured routines of modern life, our brains evolved to thrive in dynamic and unpredictable environments. Throughout human history, our ancestors faced myriad challenges and obstacles, from navigating changing weather conditions to evading predators. In response to these demands, our brains evolved to be highly adaptable, constantly learning and innovating to ensure survival.

Today, however, many aspects of our environment are vastly different from those encountered by our ancestors. The artificiality of modern lifestyles, with their predictable routines and limited variability, may not fully engage the brain's capacity for learning and adaptation. As a result, we may find ourselves craving novelty and stimulation, seeking out opportunities to challenge our minds and reignite the spark of curiosity that drives learning and growth.

In essence, while it may be easier to stick to familiar routines, actively engaging in new learning experiences is essential for maintaining the health and vitality of our brains. By embracing novelty, challenging ourselves, and fostering a mindset of lifelong learning, we can harness the full potential of our cognitive abilities and lead richer, more fulfilling lives.

Chapter 7: How Our Brains Work

Countless natural forces sculpted our brains and bodies over an incomprehensible span of time.

All species with skulls share both ancient and modern brain regions, from the old brainstem to the relatively newer cerebrum, each housing billions of neurons. Despite being separated by evolutionary time, these regions must cooperate by transmitting signals from the older parts to the newer parts and vice versa.

The dictionary defines the cerebellum as the part of the brain that coordinates and regulates muscular activity. So, which part of our brains generates muscular activity?

The cerebellum does more than just fine-tune our physical movements; it actually generates all of them by executing prelearned programs that we installed when we first acquired our motor skills. Activities like balancing, walking, running, and talking are all examples of prelearned tasks or routines. Repetition sends the same signals along the same pathways to the same neurons, strengthening these connections with each repetition until they become automatic or self-sustaining. Most physical tasks are performed without conscious thought because it is unnecessary. The routines run automatically, producing intricate muscle contractions.

Every word we speak triggers a distinct routine that we develop while learning our language.

We've all seen or set up rows of small rectangular blocks called dominoes. In these setups, only the first block needs to be knocked over to create a self-sustaining chain reaction. Once triggered, the purpose is to watch these routines as they run, but they will continue from start to finish regardless of whether we observe them or not.

The number and complexity of these routines are limited only by the number of dominoes, the available space, and the time required to build them.

Similarly, nature has been constructing our brains for hundreds of millions of years, using billions of neurons. Unlike dominoes, our brains are capable of three-dimensional growth, allowing for a vast and intricate network of routines and processes.

We build millions of routines over our lifetime, each one corresponding to a specific memory or task.

Imagine a new type of domino that stands back up shortly after being knocked over. These dominos would resemble our neurons, which can recharge and send the same signal again after a brief period. Routines built with these new dominos could be run repeatedly whenever necessary, and once constructed, each routine would run the same way each time.

A routine could be designed where the last block hits the first, creating a continuous, self-sustaining loop that runs indefinitely. Additionally, two complex routines could be constructed so that the last block of the first routine hits the first block of the second routine, and then the last block of the second routine hits the first block of the first routine. This setup would allow the first routine to run and then trigger the second, and the second to run and then trigger the first. Thus, the two routines merge into one larger, self-sustaining, automatically alternating routine.

The first routine involves the contraction of muscles to inhale, while the second involves the contraction of muscles to exhale. Similar routines can be constructed to handle other repetitive tasks, such as walking or running, among many others.

We begin constructing these routines automatically shortly after birth, and this process continues as we learn and experience new things. A new routine is formed for every memory we create, resulting in a vast number of routines built over our lifetime. However, this quantity pales in comparison to the multitude of routines already installed in our brains from birth.

For instance, we salivate when we see or smell food because a routine passed down from common ancestors was constructed in our brains while we were still developing in the womb. This innate knowledge also explains why beavers instinctively know how to build dams and why birds instinctively know how to build nests.

The majority of the routines in our brains are ancient, residing in the older regions that predate the human species by millions of years. Evolving over such an extensive period has endowed these regions with remarkable speed and efficiency. In contrast, the newer outer regions are comparatively slower and more prone to errors.

This division between the older and newer regions of our brain contributes to our perception of two distinct realms: the conscious and the subconscious. We often simplify complex processes into two distinct categories to facilitate understanding, as seen in the classic fight or flight response.

Our brains make countless instantaneous decisions, drawing upon ancient capabilities such as the ability to recognize objects, places, colors and to experience emotions like fear. These functions have been honed over millions of years of evolution, long predating the emergence of the human species.

Describing concepts in words, a skill unique to humans and managed by much more recent areas of our brain is often unnecessary. This is evident in cases where individuals with brain injuries can recognize an object but struggle to articulate its name.

Our languages are relatively recent constructs, artificial creations of human societies. While we can certainly think without speaking, our thoughts are inherently constrained by the words within our vocabulary. Consequently, our interpretations of the world around us are limited to the words we have available. For instance, the sky may appear blue to us, but this perception is exclusive to our species.

It's common for us to arrive at conclusions automatically, often without conscious thought. Many of our physical movements and thoughts are generated instantly, which can be advantageous but also problematic.

When a physical task or decision is made instantly, it's typically the result of processing by the older part of our brain, which has handled similar situations before. Conversely, the slower, more uncomfortable process of devising something new or different is the domain of the newer parts of our brain.

Each individual constructs their own reality through a lifetime of experiences. Our identities and understanding of the world are shaped by the teachings and influences we encounter over many years. We interpret everything through the lens of the words we have learned.

Neuroplasticity, the brain's ability to reorganize and form new neural connections, occurs automatically and continuously throughout our lives. This process gradually builds what we perceive as reality or consciousness by associating specific words with our experiences over time.

The ability to articulate our deepest feelings, thoughts, and emotions to ourselves and others creates the illusion of reality and consciousness. Language empowers us to explain, interpret, and perceive every aspect of our lives, shaping our understanding of the world around us.

These concepts are unique to the brains of a single species. Inadvertently, by developing the ability to communicate, we've distanced ourselves from the natural environment that gave rise to us. This transition has led to both remarkable achievements and profound challenges. For the first time in history, a relatively recent species has permanently altered its own natural evolution.

Our brains, much like our bodies, operate automatically. As we stand, signals from our senses are automatically routed to trigger the appropriate routines to maintain balance and correct any imbalances. However, when attempting something new, such as roller skating, our newer brain regions come into play. Initially, as we stumble and fall, these automatic routines don't exist, but neuroplasticity quickly kicks in, creating new pathways. With enough repetition, balancing on skates becomes easier, akin to our natural sense of balance. Eventually, the task becomes so effortless that we may tire or become bored, as what was once a challenging endeavor becomes second nature, with little engagement from the conscious part of our brain.

This is how our brains filter out repetitive sounds and smells: the same signals from our senses enter our brain but are automatically directed to trigger established routines. Initially, all signals from our senses enter the older parts of our brain, as it is structured that way and only allows necessary information to proceed further. Only novel signals are granted access to the newer regions of our brains. However, through repetition, new experiences become familiar, blurring the distinction between old and new. Consequently, we often grow tired or bored of repeating the same activities or encountering the same sensations that once elicited excitement. Over time, familiarity breeds disinterest, as the conscious part of our brain perceives little novelty or stimulation.

Consider a group of people who have been cleaning fish for years. They efficiently clean ten fish in the time it would take most of us to clean one, all while engaging in conversations and sharing laughter. Their routine has become so ingrained that it requires little conscious effort, allowing them to multitask effortlessly.

In essence, we've brought this upon ourselves. Our bodies and brains were not designed for the artificial world we've created. Our societies and environments, shaped by human innovation, often promote physical inactivity and repetitive routines, which run counter to our natural inclinations and capabilities.

We often find ourselves sedentary for hours, whether in front of screens or behind the wheel, only to realize that we need to incorporate exercise into our routines. However, our response to this realization often falls into a predictable pattern: we walk the same path in the park, wear the same shoes, or engage in the same repetitive exercises at the gym. This repetition limits our range of movement to a few predictable actions, neglecting other parts of our bodies that require attention. Paradoxically, while we believe we are preventing physical decay, we are actually perpetuating it.

Human potential knows no bounds, and we are all capable of achieving remarkable feats. Yet, without consciously challenging ourselves to explore new activities and experiences, we remain confined to the familiar. Neuroplasticity, the brain's remarkable ability to reorganize and form new connections, only activates when necessary. By adhering to the same daily routines in familiar settings, we fail to stimulate this essential process. Consequently, just as our bodies atrophy from lack of use, our brains also deteriorate when deprived of new challenges and experiences.

Our brains evolved in response to the dynamic challenges of an ever-changing natural environment, a process that has sustained our species for the vast majority of its existence.

However, until we gain a deeper understanding of the intricate workings of our brains, we are destined to repeat the mistakes of our past. The original, ancient parts of our brains wield considerable influence over our thoughts and actions, shaping our perceptions based on interpretations rooted in survival instincts. These primal regions operate swiftly and powerfully, guiding our responses to stimuli in ways that have been honed over millennia.

Conversely, the newer, slower regions of our brains are better equipped to navigate novel and unfamiliar experiences. These regions are capable of processing the complexities of new information and perceptions, albeit with discomfort and uncertainty.

In essence, our brain's evolutionary heritage influences how we interpret and respond to the world around us. Only by comprehending the intricacies of this organ can we hope to transcend the patterns of our past and embrace new possibilities for growth and adaptation.

About the Book

Imagine a revolutionary approach to achieving and maintaining a better level of Health and Fitness accessible to individuals of any age and ability. This method involves engaging in direct physical movements with a constant variation in direction intensities, durations, and speeds. Unlike traditional exercises, it minimizes repetition, eliminating the concept of reps or sets.

The uniqueness lies in the absence of predetermined movements or routines; instead, participants spontaneously create movements on the go, tailoring them to their own pace and intensity levels to align with their abilities. The flexibility in intensity control allows for gradual initiation, enabling individuals to elevate intensity based on personal preferences and physical capacity incrementally.

What sets this approach apart is its adaptability to any environment, at any time, and in any position, without the need for specialized equipment. Participants can utilize their surroundings creatively, incorporating anything and everything available for an engaging and dynamic fitness experience.

Steven never dreamed he would try to write a book on health and fitness, but he had to do something. The knowledge he gained over years of research gave him a new perspective on how our minds and bodies work and how this is causing some disturbing trends in our current society. This book is meant to try to illustrate to the readers the intricately complex automated systems of our minds and bodies that go on constantly without our knowledge to get us through our everyday lives. Our health and well-being depend significantly on many of these automated systems running together, often, and properly. A problem with one system can lead to problems with all systems. Our bodies and minds were designed to function the way they do by intricate natural forces over an incomprehensible period of time.

Made in the USA
Columbia, SC
17 December 2024

49619842R00041